PROSTRATE CARE - NATURAL REMEDIES FOR PROSTRATE PROBLEMS : URINE RETENTION AND OTHER RELATED PROSTRATE DIORDERS IN MEN –NUTRITIONAL REMEDIES Series VI

REVISED

2016

T.A. Shobukola

CONTENTS

DEDICATION

I dedicate this book to the Glory and honour of the almighty God, The Creator and , Giver of life and The great Physician. I thank and adore Him for the inspiration and determination given for this little effort . May His name be praised forever.

ACKNOWLEDGEMENT

 I wish to express my heart-felt appreciation to all those who had contributed in one way or the other to the success of this project; especially authors whose works are cited or quoted in this book. I also glorify God for the Book of books, The holy Bible.

FOREWORD

This passage in The Word of God, Ps 139 :14 - **" I will praise Thee ,for I am fearfully and wonderfully made: marvelous are Thy works; and that my soul knoweth right well. "**- sums up the wonderful and intricately complex nature of man as created by God to meet all forms of health challenges of life.

This is also succinctly expressed by George Malkmus and others in the book "Hallelujah Diet" where   he writes that every person is born with more wondrously self-healing mechanism , built right into their bodies than you could ever find in a hospital ". He writes further , " ….our brilliant Designer installed…..a genetic code ….. complete with Painkillers for emergencies, Antibiotics for infections, Dressings for wounds and Micro-surgery wards , capable of replacing damaged cells with brand new ones."

 We only need to " eat right and live well " to enable the body helps itself to actualize this innate self- healing mechanism in the body.

Eating right entails eating good and functional foods which are foods that go far beyond just providing basic nutrition but also perform specific medicinal effects in the body .

Foods can heal in ways drugs never can this is because drugs can only relieve the symptoms of disease, but rarely cure the underlying condition the way foods can. The reason being that   our bodies evolved over millions of years to thrive on foods. Foods are nature's way to repair, restore and rejuvenate. They heal the body without dangerous side effects.

It had been said that Food, or lack of it, is the main cause of the vast majority of our health problems, and therefore food is also the solution.

 This is further corroborated by a saying in natural medicine: "For every disease known to man, there's a country where it virtually doesn't exist."- The Japanese have lower rates of heart disease. East Indians rarely get Alzheimer's. What makes the difference is Diet- Food.

It isthereforein line with the foregoing that all the recommendations in this book are food-based since God in His infinite wisdom and love for mankind   had made it possible for man to know which particular food is good for which parts of the body.

INTRODUCTION

The prostate gland is an important part of every man's reproductive system . It is located in the pelvic area, just below the outlet of the bladder, in front of the rectum of a man . It encircles the upper part of the urethra, the tube that empties urine from the bladder. It also plays an important role in production of semen .

The strategic importance of the gland therefore makes it imperative for all men to take adequate care to maintain a healthy prostrate gland.

This book sets out to enumerate the best ways to maintain a healthy prostrate, by listing the different possible prostrate health challenges and the corresponding natural remedies to combat them without resorting to drugs with their attendant adverse effects which most of the time are worse than the problems they are expected to solve.

CHAPTER ONE

What is the Prostate Gland?

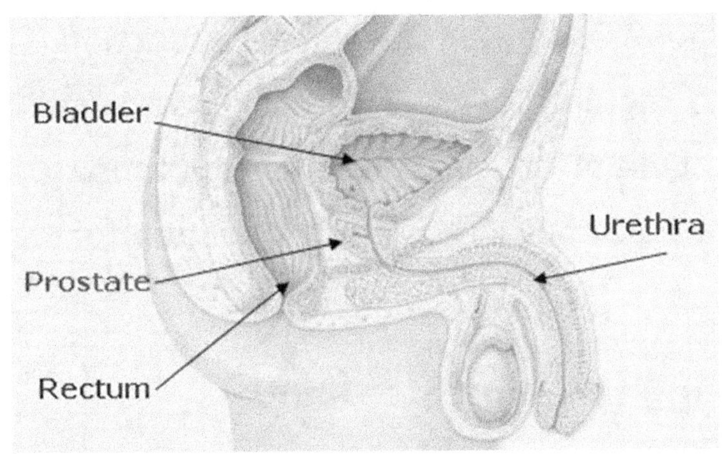

The prostate gland is a walnut-sized gland located in the pelvic area, just below the outlet of the bladder and in front of the rectum of a man .It encircles the upper part of the urethra, which is the tube that empties urine from the bladder. The prostate gland is only present in males..A normal prostrate gland naturally causes no problems for urine flow.

The healthy human prostate is slightly larger than a walnut and although it is called a gland, since it is made of two lobes completely surrounded by an outer tissue layer; the term "organ" may be a more fitting description.

It is a part of every man's reproductive system and it requires male hormones, like testosterone, to function properly, helping to regulate bladder controland normal sexual functioning. One of the prostate's functions is to nourish semen, the fluid that keeps sperm healthy for fertilization

Conditions affecting the Prostate Gland

Risk factors for prostate cancer include age, race, nationality, family history, genes, obesity, exercise, smoking and diet.

Prostate problem is a sad fact for men growing older, as most of the men over 60 years of age (and some in their 50s) develop one or other types of prostate problem symptoms.

When a man is younger, the prostate is walnut-sized, but as he ages, the prostate can grow to about the size of an egg.

Regardless of age, keeping your prostate healthy is key to supporting optimal urine flow, vitality, and a healthy sex drive.

CHAPTER TWO

The three most common disorders of the prostrate are:

- ➢ Enlargement of the prostate called Benign Prostatic Hyperplasia (BPH),
- ➢ Prostatitis, an inflammatory infection; and

- ➢ Prostate cancer.

Ignoring prostate problems, or leaving it untreated, as some are wont to do, can make it get progressively worse, become more painful, and caneventually lead to dangerous complications, such as bladder and kidney infections.

Enlarged Prostate (BPH):

BPH is the most common prostate problem for men, older than 50, Since the prostate has the propensity to grow once manhood is reached.

It said to be so common that some physicians erroneously consider it a normal consequence of aging in males.

With ageing, the body gets heavier and loses its flexibility. This puts greater pressure on the pelvis and increases the vulnerability of the prostate gland.
Prolonged period of sitting, as in certain sedentary occupations, also increases the pressure on the pelvic region, resulting in congestion of the tissues in and around the prostate gland .The prostate gland slowly enlarges and tends to expand in an area that does not expand with it, thereby causing pressure on the urethra,this causes the prostate gland to press against the urethra like a clamp on a garden hose ,the bladder wall becomes thicker and irritable and begins to contract even when it contains small amounts of urine, leading to more frequent urination and other urinary problems like a weak bladder, bladder or kidney infections, complete blockage of urine flow , and kidney failure.

It should be noted that an enlarged prostate is not a sign of prostate cancer and is not life-threatening, but it can be extremely uncomfortable with painful or troublesome symptoms.

Some Symptoms include:

> difficulty urinating

> frequent urination, especially at night

> difficulty starting urination

> inability to empty the bladder

➢ weak urinary stream,

➢ a dribble of urine despite the urgent need to urinate
> a burning sensation when urinating

> uncontrolled dribbling after urination

> pain behind the scrotum

> painful ejaculation

2. **Prostatitis**: .

Prostatitis isan inflammatory infection of the prostate gland
,

 a condition that involves inflammation of the prostate gland in
men.It can either be bacterial or non-bacterial in nature.

The nonbacterial Prostatitis (chronic pelvic pain
syndrome) is the most common, but least understood,
form of prostatitis. Found in men of any age from the
late teens on, the symptoms go away and then return
without warning, and may be inflammatory or non-
inflammatory.

Depending on the type of prostatitis, the condition can cause urinary problems and pain, as well as fever, nausea, blood in the urine or semen and frequent bladder infections.

It is most commonly caused by an infectionwhen bacteria from the urethra travels to the prostate, and can cause addition symptoms.

Some of the symptoms are

- ➢ muscle and joint pain,
- ➢ Fever, chills and flulike symptoms
- ➢ Pain in the prostate gland, scrotum, or lower back
- ➢ Urinary frequency and
- ➢ blood–tinged urine
- ➢ Painful ejaculation
- ➢ involuntary discharge of urine.

3Prostate Cancer:

It is the Cancer affecting the prostate gland. It is the most common cancer in some men.

Prostate cancer grows slowly and may not spread for many years.

Symptoms include:

- *difficulty starting urine flow.*
- pain during urination.
- loss of weight and appetite,
- blood in urine,
- painful ejaculation.

Symptoms of advanced prostate cancer include:

- Dull, incessant deep pain or stiffness in the pelvis, lower back, ribs or upper thighs; arthritic pain in the bones of those areas
- Loss of weight and appetite
- Fatigue
- Nausea
- Vomiting

Some common symptoms of the different types of prostrate disorders.

The different prostate gland problems sometimes have similar symptoms. For example, one man with prostatitis and another with BPH may both have a frequent, urgent need to urinate. A man with BPH may have trouble beginning a stream of urine; another may have to urinate frequently at night. Also a man in the early stages of prostate cancer may have no symptoms at all.

- Sensation of not emptying your bladder completely after you have finished urinating.
- Frequent urination (consistently in intervals of less than 2 hours and / or multiple times during the night).
- Interrupted urination (you have to stop and start several times during urination).
- Difficulty in postponing urination.
- Weak or limited urinary stream.
- Pushing and straining to begin urination.
- A burning pain during urination.
- Pain in lower back, in the area between the testicles and anus, in the lower belly or upper thighs, or above the pubic area. Pain may be worse during bowel movement.
- Reduced ability to gain and hold erection.
- Weak ejaculation.
- Dissatisfaction with sexual performance.
- Some pain during or after ejaculation.

- Pain in the tip of the penis.
- Fever and chills.
- Loss of appetite.

It should be noted that one prostate problem does not lead to another. For example, having prostatitis or an enlarged prostate does not increase the chance for prostate cancer. It is true that some men with prostate cancer also have BPH, but the two conditions are not automatically linked. Most men with BPH do not develop prostate cancer. But because the early symptoms for both conditions could be the same, a health practitioner would need to evaluate them. It is however possible to have more than one condition at a time.

CHAPTER THREE

NATURAL REMEDIES

Earlydetection is of great deal in treating any prostrate problem Once any of the symptoms is noted the treatment should commence immediately.
Clinical studies have been performed that show the benefits of taking natural supplements to prevent and or treat enlarged prostate problem; showing that herbs can be used to treat enlarged prostate symptoms effectively and often much more gently. Many of such herbs have been used by men for centuries with positive results.

> ➢ It had been shown thatGhent University Hospital in Belgium conducted a study in 2004 which showed selenium, **lycopene, saw palmetto and vitamin E** combined had a positive impact on hormonal charged prostate growth.

➢ This study suggested a holistic approach to managing prostate health, which includes the use of natural supplements.

Equally, records confirm that the Institute of Clinical Medicine at National Cheng Kung University in Taiwan indicated that *oil* derived ***from pumpkin seeds*** can prevent prostate enlargement.

In the same vein,Duke University concluded that When flaxseed is combined with other nutrients it can have a positive impact on overall prostate health.

The University of Maryland Medical Center also noted that Stinging nettle is a commonly used botanical remedy in the treatment of BPH and that when combined with certain other herbs, may be helpful in treating BPH-related symptoms, including low urine flow, incomplete bladder voiding and the persistent urge to urinate.For prostate support, stinging nettle extract capsules or tablets can be taken at a dose of 80 mg per day, according to the University of Maryland Medical Center.

Orthodox Medicine Approach:

Western medicine relies on aggressive and costly prescription drugs and prohibitively-expensive surgery to deal with problems related to prostate and reproductive disorders.

These methods generally address only the symptoms of prostate disorder and not the underlying causes. As soon as the drug is stopped, the problem returns! These prescription drugs often result in unwanted and more dangerous side effects.

The medical options, through the use of drugs can cause as much concern as the original symptoms. The combined side effects include :

* breast tenderness and enlargement,
* decreased sex drive,
* difficulty getting an erection,
* dizziness,
* fainting,

❖ headache,

❖ heart failure,

❖ increased ejaculatory dysfunction,

❖ lightheadedness,

❖ nasal congestion,

❖ retrograde ejaculation (ejaculation back into the bladder),

❖ sudden drop in blood pressure,

❖ tiredness,

❖ upper respiratory tract infection

Danger of prostrate removal:

Some side effects of Prostrate removal include :

> Loss of libido

> Full sexual dysfunction

> Urine incontinence.

> *bleeding,*

> *blood clotting,*

> *damage to other nearby organs*

- ➢ Impotence is a rather common side effect

- ➢ hair loss,

- ➢ and even death.

Speaking on prostate surgery an expert had once said , "While many doctors think immediately of eliminating the problem, they think very little of the treatment's devastating side effects that seriously diminish the patient's quality of life. And, for the 40,000 American men who have their prostates removed each year, 35 percent of the men afflicted find themselves dealing with the return of the disease within just five years."

Prostate Specific Antigen -PSA

PSA refers to prostate-specific antigen. PSA is a protein produced in the prostate gland. A high PSA usually indicates the presence of prostate cancer. Fortunately, there are natural treatments that help lower PSA levels, and prevent prostate cancer; Herbs like saw palmetto lower PSA. Green tea and other herbal blends are said to lower PSA levels as well.

Commenting on the PSA ,in his writing titled "Exposed! The Prostate Cancer Scam of the Century" , Dr. William Campbell Douglass the author of the ' FREE health newsletter' who was nick-named " medicine's most popular mythbuster" , because he had made it his mission to reveal the surprisingly inexpensive and easy road to real health - to the chagrin of pharmaceutical companies and surgeons everywhere , wrote " Strong words, I know - but time and again science has proven that the prostate specific antigen (PSA) screening is unreliable at best, downright dangerous at worst. Even the Journal of the American Medical Association (JAMA) spoke out in opposition to the PSA, saying: "A blood test for prostate cancer may lead to more problems than it is worth."

He wrote further, ' The PSA is not "prostate-specific" as the name indicates: A bad cold or other form of infection may cause an elevation of what's supposed to be the "prostate-specific" antigen.It had been said that high levels of PSA do not always mean prostate cancer is present.

 Can you imagine deciding to have prostate surgery - something that will likely leave you impotent and incontinent for the rest of your life - based on such an unreliable test? I know I can't. But thousands of men who don't know any better do it every single day.

 In conclusion, he said "Mainstream medicine's solution: Slash and Burn!

-      It's true. And it's sad, too. The most common form of modern prostate surgery involves jamming a quarter-inch-thick pipe half a foot or so up your urethra (yep, you read that right), then frying your prostate with a hot wire loop. Not a lot of fun." There's no denying it, the PSA test is worthless.

It is   therefore highly advisable **to adopt the natural option to shrink** the prostrate and avoid the removal which is the common medical approach for the treatment .

 Some natural approach for treating enlarged prostate problem include :
- ➤ **following a low-fat diet,**
- ➤ **maintaining a healthy lifestyle**
  - **Reduce your stress** –

    Most people know stress can have a profound effect on health. Scientists have shown links between stress and less-than-optimal prostate health. Look for ways to relieve stress in your life such as using the Emotional Freedom Technique (EFT).
  - **Relax your muscles** – Muscle tension can impact your prostate health. A regular exercise program can do wonders to help reduce muscle tension and trigger a more positive attitude and mood
  - **Boost your lymphatic system** – Your lymphatic system is responsible for clearing your body of waste and plays an essential role in your prostate vitality. Regular

exercise and drinking adequate amounts of pure, fresh water can help flush waste and toxins out of your body.

• **Cleanse your body on the inside** – The build-up of toxins inside the body can have a profound effect on your overall health, including the prostate health as well.

• **Revitalize love and sexual activity** –. A healthy sex life is food for the prostate. Also, nurturing your personal relationships and love can help reduce stress as well.

Research has shown sexual activity and a high ejaculation frequency are linked to better prostate health later in life by helping support the body's natural detoxification functions. Frequent ejaculation may help act as one of your body's natural detoxification functions for your prostate glands.

CHATER FOUR

NUTRIRITIONAL/HERBAL REMEDIES

A relief for nagging, constant symptoms of an enlarged prostate, can be found in going back to the basics byfollowing a very simple approach .

One of such basic and natural routines that can be employed to reduce the symptoms involves just taking a daily supplement , few diet changes, some basic exercise and other lifestyle modifications.

Herbal prostate treatment options are gaining a lot of popularity lately. With clinical studies supporting their results, this gentler approach to prevention and symptom relief is providing a solution for many men.

There are a number of reasons why natural / herbal prostate treatment options are proving so beneficial. Firstly, the ingredients used in herbal prostate treatments are natural and work gently in the body without any adverse side effects.

Secondly a number of different natural substances have come under thescientific scrutiny of researchers and stood out well as natural potent remedies for prostrate challenges.
Some of the most notable ones include:

Lycopene

Lycopene is a compound that gives certain fruits and vegetables their color.
It is a carotenoid and one of the antioxidants said to have shown reduced incidence of cancer.

Clinical studies have strongly indicated that lycopene can have a large impact on protecting prostate health. This particular natural supplement can be very useful in preventing prostate problems and it can assist in reducing prostate growth if issues are already present. This substance has been shown to be quite useful in not only treating and preventing age-related prostate enlargement, but also prostate cancer, as well.

Some fruits and veggies which contain this carotenoidare:

Pink Guava:

Guavas with pink flesh are loaded with lycopene

Watermelon .

Every cup of watermelon is packed with great amount of lycopene. It is also an excellent source of vitamin C and a very good source of vitamin A. It is rich in potassium, magnesium, thiamin, vitamin B6, copper and manganese.

The Amish use watermelon tea to flush out the system and help with bladder problems and prostate problems.

The seeds are equally effective. Add boiling water to 1/8 cup of fresh watermelon seeds and allow to cool , strained and taken as tea every day .

Lemon juice

Forego all solid foods and subsist on water, mixed with a little lemon juice, for two or three days. The water may be taken cold or hot and it should be taken every hour or so, during wake-up hours. This will greatly increase the flow of urine

Horsetail

For an enlarged prostate, an infusion of Horsetail can help a good deal: It is a strong diuretic, increasing urine flow and helping the bladder toempty itself completely . It is also astringent and anti- inflammatory, toning the swollen membranes.

Persimmon

The Japanese persimmon is another excellent source of vitamin A and a very good sources of manganese and fiber. It contains reasonable amount of lycopene. It is also rich in vitamins E, K and B6 and the minerals copper and potassium.

Grapefruit

Pink and red grapefruits are excellent sources of the two potent antioxidants—vitamins A and C. They also contain fiber, potassium, thiamin, vitamin B6 and pantothenic acid. Every cup is packed with lycopene.

Apricot

Another fruit that's brimming with vitamins A and C is apricot. It is also rich in vitamins E and K, fiber, copper and manganese and contains half the potassium content of bananas.

Papaya

Considered as one of the most nutritious fruits, papaya is chockfull of vitamin C. It is also packed with vitamin A, foliate, potassium and fiber

Bell Pepper

One cup of chopped red bell pepper is packed with three times the daily needed value of vitamin C and almost 100% of vitamin A. It is also rich in vitamins E and B6 as well as foliate and fiber.

Tomatoes.

 Studies have shown that a little servings of tomatoes (including cooked tomatoes) a week can help in reducing the risk of prostate cancer by half. These red orbs are full of lycopene

Red Cabbage

Red cabbage is an excellent source of vitamin C. Every one cup of shredded cabbage contains high percentage of the daily needed value of this vitamin. It is also packed with vitamins K and B6, and manganese and contains good quantity of lycopene.

Asparagus

Although lycopene is more commonly found in red fruits and veggies, it has also been found in cooked asparagus . Asparagus is considered as one of the most nutritious vegetables ;being an excellent source of vitamins A, C and K and the fertility-promoting mineral–foliate. It's also a good source of more than a dozen other nutrients.

Stinging nettle

The stinging nettle plant is a herbaceous perennial. Today, stinging nettle is among the best herbs for enlarged prostate, used in conjunction with saw palmetto and pygeum, the herb may reduce the bothersome side effects of enlarged prostate, such as urinary retention and urinary urgency, according to " Medline Plus".

Stinging nettle, an abundant, prickly plant found in Europe ,parts of Asia and Africa is also a medicinal herb to treat anemia, inflammation of the urinary tract and other health complications. Topically, the herb is a remedy for sprains, joint pain and insect bites.

 For BPH, the herb is used alone or in conjunction with saw palmetto and pygeum to help reduce the symptoms of enlarged prostate and shrink the prostate by increasing testosterone in the body.

 Other uses for stinging nettle include impotence, allergies, migraines and rheumatoid arthritis.

Saw palmetto, or Serenoa repens, , also known as the American dwarf palm or cabbage tree is used to treat an enlarged prostate. It is a palm native to the southeastern United States and

Caribbea, found growing naturally in the tropical climate from South Carolina to Florida. Saw palmetto is a small plant used in ancient herbal medicine as a tonic, expectorant and antiseptic

The herb is effective in shrinking the prostate and relieving the symptoms of enlarged prostate. According to Medline Plus, the herb is the most popular treatment for BPH, more commonly used in Europe. Its effectiveness in BPH may be due to its multiple actions against an enlarging prostate.

Saw palmetto is best known for its use as a herbal remedy for BPH, but it is also used to treat prostatitis symptoms, says the University of Michigan Health System.

"According to laboratory studies, saw palmetto contains constituents that act to reduce swelling and inflammation," the University of Michigan explained.

The University of Maryland Medical Center advised taking 160 mg capsules of saw palmetto supplement twice daily to help treat non-bacterial prostatitis..

The extract of the berries of this plant has been shown to work as well and better than prescription drugs in improving urinary flow rates and reducing the symptoms of BPH, such as urinary hesitancy and weak flow. The extract works by altering certain hormone levels, thus reducing prostate enlargement.

 Palmetto extracts capsules can be purchased at the health food stores.

Pumpkin seeds

These seeds are used to treat urination problems caused by an enlarged benign prostate. Pumpkin seeds are loaded with zinc and have plenty of diuretic properties which help to repair and build immune system.

The seeds act as a rich source of unsaturated fatty acid, which are vital to the health of the prostate. About 50 gm seeds are to be taken daily either in cooked food or powdered. . The seeds may be taken in the form of powder , sprinkled over cooked vegetables or mixed with wheat flour. They can also be taken in the form of a paste made with honey.

Pumpkin seeds are used by German doctors to treat difficult urination that accompanies an enlarged prostate that is not cancerous.

The tastiest way to enjoy pumpkin seeds is to eat them plain, after removing the shells .

You can also take as tea; Crush a handful of fresh seeds , place in the tea jar and fill with boiling water. Let cool to room temperature, strain and drink a pint as tea, a day.

Enlarged prostate supplements very often contain this ingredient. It has been shown to help maintain prostate health, reduce symptoms and even prevent them.

The seed is available in capsule form in health stores .

Goldenseal

Another very useful and powerful way of treating swollen prostate is by using Goldenseal. It does not only heals the urinary tract, but also helps to bring down the swelling of a swollen prostate gland.

Bee Pollen

 Bee pollen is also very helpful in helping people overcome swollen prostate since it actually helps in shrinking the prostate that has become swollen.

However, it should be noted that bee pollen can only be taken in the early stages of the Prostate growth.

Pygeum,

It is a herbal extracted from the evergreen tree ,PrunusAfricana, which is native to Africa.

Among the Zulu people of Africa, the herb was a treatment for BPH, and for other related issues. it is a remedy for urinary tract problems.It is an aphrodisiac and had various other uses. According to Medline Plus, it is noted for significantly reducing urinary urgency, frequency and pain with urination among men with mild to moderate symptoms of BPH.

 It can be found in various formulations combining with other herbs , such as saw palmetto and stinging nettle for shrinking the prostate .They are available over-the-counter in health stores.

The bark of Pygeum,had been used for thousands of years to treat bladder disorders and urination problems associated with benign prostatic hypertrophy (BPH) ,Prostrate enlargement. African pygeum extract may help to treat both bacterial and non-bacterial prostatitis in men. It acts to reduce the urinary symptoms from prostatitis, as well as benign prostatic hyperplasia, or "BPH,"

Green Tea and Prostate Cancer?

Green tea is one of the most widely consumed beverages in the world.

Medicinally, green tea is often used to treat cardiovascular disease. It also may be helpful for cancer. In certain populations where people drink more drinks than others there appeared to be a lower level of incidence of several different types of cancers. Studies were carried out to see what type of beverage was having this positive effect in the reduction in the development of different types of cancers. The results pointed out that green tea was the positive influence that was helping prevent cancer.

Dr. Yarnell reported that in eastern Asia, where green tea consumption is very prevalent, prostate cancer rates are very low, particularly amongst the people who lead non-western lifestyles. It is shows that green tea plays a role in preventing prostate cancer.

 Also, lab tests show evidence of green tea's prostate cancer-fighting abilities.

 The Memorial Sloan-Kettering Cancer Center attributes the anti-cancer activity of green tea to its polyphenol content. Experts also pointed out that the active component in the tea leaves are believed to be catechins, a kind of antioxidant.

Green tea, with its many beneficial effects and positive safety record, may be useful adjunct to a well-rounded treatment plan for prostate cancer.

Health care professionals all agree that drinking green tea instead of coffee is healthier due to lower caffeine content and higher nutrition value.

Corn Silk

The silk from corn , is usually called mother's hair and India corn among other names It contains plant acids, Vitamins C and K along with other contents

It had been used by Amish men for generations as a remedy for the symptoms of prostate enlargement. It can be harvested when fresh corn is in season and can be shade- dried and preserved for later use, too. It is also available in capsule and tablet forms in major   health stores

It has detoxifying, relaxing and diuretic properties. It is noted for the treatment of infections of the urinary and genital systems; such as cystitis , prostatitis , enlargement of the prostrate ad other prostrate challenges.

It helps to reduce painful   and frequent urination caused by irritation of the bladder and bed wetting problems.

 For usage , put in 1 quart of water, boil, and simmer for ten minutes. Strain and drink a cup thrice a week.

Fish.

Fresh fish from the deep fights prostate cancer and tumor growth. Eating two servings a week of fish high in omega-3 oils (the good oil), such as tuna, mackerel, or salmon is recommended.

Peppermint

Peppermint herb in tea form has potent anti-bacterial and anti-fungi properties that helps in prostrate problems.

Ginger and Cayene

Other items that should be included in the diet are ginger and cayenne. These can prevent problems with the prostate gland.

Carrot and spinach

Drinking carrot juice is believed to be beneficial in this condition. You can also make a mixture of 300 ml of carrot juice and 200 ml of spinach. Drinking this will solve problems of the swollen glands.

Spices

Garlic, Turmeric, Ginger and Rosemary act as good and potent supplements for an enlarge Prostate problem.

Other foodstuffs

Experts had identified more Nigerian foodstuffs with prostate cancer chemo-preventive substances.Such foods include native pear(Ube), cloves, horseradish/Moringa oleifera, bush candle tree, wild cabbage, soursop, soya beans, chilli pepper.

Benefits of Soy

Another potent supplement for an enlarged prostate is Soy (soy milk). Hormone stability is important for good prostate health. The versatile soybean contains flavonoids, which are compounds that help the body achieve this hormonal balance. Although many vegetarian and vegan dishes contain soy and soy products, it is recommended for optimal health benefits to obtain the soy from the actual soybean or from tofu.

It has been documented that populations whose diet is based on soybeans and soy products have a lower incidence of prostate cancer. The active ingredient in soy is thought to be phytoestrogens, or plant estrogens

Benefits of Nuts and Seeds

According to Reader's Digest (Foods That Harm Foods That Heal), vitamin E has been instrumental with inflammation reduction and protection against prostate cancer. Good sources include egg yolks, wheat germ, nuts and seeds. Pumpkin seeds, flax seeds, sunflower seeds and hemp are especially helpful, as they help regulate hormones. Almonds, Brazil nuts and walnuts are low in saturated fat and contain vitamin E and other protective nutrients. Foods with anti-inflammatory properties such as ginger and onions also offer good support.

Vegetables and Fruits

Consuming vegetables and fruits plays an important role in your prostate health. Fresh fruits is beneficial for good prostate health. The natural sugar contained in them have a protective effect on the gland.

Some vegetables contain another antioxidant called sulforaphane, which is useful in reducing inflammation, repairing oxidative damage and removing carcinogens. Broccoli, cabbage and kale, are good choices of leafy, green vegetables that contain sulforaphane.

In addition to vitamins and nutrients, they contain antioxidants such as vitamin C, which promotes immune functions and decreases prostate inflammation, reports Dr. Michael Blute in the publication "Mayo Clinic on Prostate Health." Vitamin C-rich vegetables and fruits include oranges, sweet peppers, broccoli, onions, tomatoes, asparagus, grapefruit, green peas, brussels sprouts, cantaloupe, cabbage and other leafy greens. Juicing fruits and vegetables is an additional way to supply your body with nutrients that may shrink prostate inflammation.

Cranberry

Drink cranberry juice. Cranberry juice increases the acidity of urine, making the urinary tract an unwelcome environment of bacteria which cause urinary tract infections. Drinking cranberry juice four times a day, in addition to the eight glasses of water, should increase your arsenal against urinary tract infections

Whole Grains

Whole grains contain all nutritious parts of the grain, including the endosperm, germ and bran. As a result, they provide more vitamins, minerals, antioxidants and fiber than refined grains such as white flour and instant rice.

A diet rich in natural fiber may help lower your risk for prostate cancer and prostate cancer progression, according to the University of California San Francisco Medical Center.

Whole-grain foods contain nutrients that help support body functions and promote prostate health. According to the "Mayo Clinic on Prostate Health," these nutrients include niacin, thiamine, folate, biotin, iron and selenium, which may help shrink an enlarged prostate. They also contain fiber and low-fat content, which can reduce constipation and balance blood sugar levels, all of which can benefit the prostate health. Ideal whole grains to consume include cracked wheat, whole rye, spelt, millet, whole-grain pasta, whole-grain bread, brown rice, wild rice, buckwheat , oats,barley, brown rice, wild rice, millet and air-popped popcorn

Legumes, such as split-peas, beans and lentils, provide rich amounts of fiber and protein. They also provide saturated fat and cholesterol-free alternatives to fatty meats Nutritious legume-based dishes include split-pea soup, lentil soup, steamed soybeans and low-fat vegetarian chili.

CHAPTER FIVE

SUPPLIMENTS

Most people know about common antioxidants present in fruits and vegetables such as Vitamins A, C, E . Practically every plant in the world contains unique types of antioxidants with varying levels of potency..

It is well known that consuming sufficient types of vegetables and fruits is very difficult because of their non-availability. Some of these are marigolds, saw palmetto, red clover, nettle root, passion flower, algae and gingko biloba, to mention a few.

Therefore the best solution may be in food supplements which are readily available in health stores and supermarkets.

Some helpful natural supplements which are very potent for the treatment of prostate gland problems :

Selenium .

This is what is called every man's "must-have mineral." Its power to support the immune system is remarkable. It is especially helpful and essential for good prostate health. As with lycopene, studies consistently show that men with higher levels of selenium have healthier prostates.

It is easily found in some food items like Okro, onion, Wheat germ and brewer's yeast, wheat germ, tuna, herring and other seafood and shellfish, beef liver and kidney, eggs, sunflower and sesame seeds, cashews, Brazil nuts, mushrooms, garlic, onions, etc.

These days, getting sufficient selenium from your diet looks harder hence the importance of supplementing.

Omega-3 Fatty Acids

Omega-3 fatty acids, or omega-3s, are healthy, essential fats that must be obtained from food. Omega-3 fats may reduce risk for prostate cancers, according to the University of Maryland Medical Center. They may also help alleviate inflammation associated with prostatitis and other prostate-related health conditions.

Rich amounts of omega-3 fats are found in coldwater fish, such as mackerel, Alaskan salmon, lake trout, herring, sardines and albacore tuna. Walnuts, ground flaxseed, flaxseed oil and canola oil provide similar omega-3 benefits. The University of Maryland Medical Center recommends coldwater fish at least twice per week for optimum wellness

Zinc

Zinc is a real "man's mineral." It is really a sexual health booster which is essential for maximum prostate health!

It is a vital nutrient contained in healthy prostate and reproductive fluids.

It is aid that the semen has 100 times more zinc than the blood while the prostate has the highest concentration of zinc in the body.Itmaximizes testosterone production and extends the life of testosterone in the bloodstream .

It is found in such food as cabbage, Spinach, Fish, Apples, Beet root ,Melon , Pumpkin seed in the shell, oysters, beans, and nuts .

Vitamin E

Vitamin Eis one of the most effective and versatile antioxidants on the planet. Together with other elements, vitamin E targets dangerous free radicals and provides the prostate with a shield of protection ,sheltering it from the ravages of aging, oxidation and external threats.

Dozens of ||studies over the last two decades show the remarkable power of vitamin E and its ability to promote prostate health for a lifetime. It even helps reduce androgens (male hormones), which you need to keep at normal levels for a healthy prostate.

Vitamin E gives the manhood a boost too!Vitamin E helps maintain the lining of the blood vessels . It is well-known known that having healthy blood vessel flexibility is central to achieving and maintaining an erection.

Vitamin D: This is the main player in prostate health, without any question ; it is such an important element to overall health. The best source is sunlight .

Always consult with your healthcare professional to determine the optimal dose of Vitamin D to best support your health.

Vitamin K2: This is only available from bacterial fermentation. Vitamin K2 is the only form of vitamin K that has been shown to help promote prostate health.

Calcium and Magnesium: This had been shown to be essential for an-optimal prostate health . Magnesium is available in some natural foods ,like leafy green vegetables,whole grains, nut such as cashew , in fruits like figs and also in sweet corn, shrimps ,milk and sun flower seed.

Vitamins C and B6

Doses of Vitamin C and Vitamin B6 are some of the best supplements for prostate health. They make urination easier and prevent swelling.

CHAPTER SIX

There are some good and helpful measures that are necessary for maintaining a healthy prostate.

 To maintain a good prostate health the following should be carefully avoided ;

   ✓ Excess sexual acts,

✓ Irregularity in eating and drinking,

✓ Long periods of sitting on a chair . The use of a relaxing chair which helps in reducing pressure on the prostate is highly recommended.

✓ **alcohol intake**

Alcohol depletes both zinc and vitamin B6 (which is necessary for zinc absorption)

Studies have also shown that beer can raise prolactin levels in the body, which in turn can eventually lead to prostate enlargement

✓ **Avoid the use of caffeine.**

Stimulating drinks such as soda, black tea, coffee and alcoholic beverages should be limited.

Foods to Avoid

Certain foods are thought to contribute to prostate cancer and should be avoided.

Low-fat Diet

The University of California at San Francisco recommends a low-fat diet for prostate cancer. They suggest that one should aim to get 20 percent of the total calories from fat. Less than 10 percent should come from saturated fat. Trans fat should also be restricted

Avoid mayonnaise, butter, baked goods, regular salad dressings, margarine, fried foods, cheese and processed foods.

Red meat and dairy products should be restricted for prostate cancer. The University of California at San Francisco suggested that an increased consumption of red meat and dairy is related to an increased risk of metastatic prostate cancer. Red meat and dairy products contain saturated fat which is the main reason why they should be restricted. If you do choose to eat some dairy, choose the fat-free or low-fat options.

Simple Sugars

Simple sugars should be avoided when following a prostate cancer diet. Avoid processed and refined grains, flours and sugars. White foods should be restricted, including breads, pastas, rice, cereal, cream sauces and cakes

Choose whole wheat or whole grain breads, pastas and cereals. Choose brown rice instead of white rice. Foods high in sugar also tend to be low in nutrients including fiber, which is why they are not recommended.

Diet Guidelines

The University of California at San Francisco developed dietary guidelines for prostate health. In addition to avoiding the food items mentioned above, one should incorporate at least eight to 10 colorful fruits and vegetables daily.

Eat healthy fats such as olive oil, salmon, trout, walnuts and soybeans. Incorporate tomato products in your diet to obtain more of the antioxidant lycopene. Finally, drink plenty of fluids

✓ Eliminate added salt and salty foods.
✓ In addition, avoid drinking liquids with or just before meals, because they dilute the digestive enzymes,

resulting in poor digestion and decreased nutrient absorption.

Adopting Healthy Lifestyle

Avoid **vigorous exercise** .Moderate exercises may help. Such exercise involves contracting the muscles around the scrotum and anus. This increases blood flow to prostate tissue and, in theory, may provide some benefit by reliefing urinary   problems and other symptoms related to fluid retention.

Regular exercise has been shown to strengthen the immune system and improve digestion, circulation, and the removal of waste matter from the body. Exercise also prevents obesity, which is a risk factor for many diseases, including cancer. Regular exercise may also reduce the risk of prostate gland enlargement.

Kidney Cleansing

Kidney cleansing is an important aspect of cleansing the prostate, as the kidneys are the primary means for the prostate to flush toxins. To cleanse the kidneys, you must be consuming sufficient water, juices, and herbal teas. Top kidney cleansing herbs include juniper, uva ursi, dandelion leaves, corn silk, parsley, and horsetail.

Although these kidney cleansing herbs are not herbs for prostate health per se, they form an important part of any comprehensive herbal prostate treatment.

Hydrotherapy treatment

Hydrotherapy is an ancient healing art that is safe and painless, requiring nothing exotic than the natural water from the tap or well.

First used by Hippocrates ,the father of medicine in the fourth century B.C. ,hydrotherapy had been a part of the healing tradition of nearly every civilization, from ancient Greek and Egypt to Rome, where virtually every public medicine was practiced at the public Baths,

Fluids

Drinking fluids, such as water, has a positive effect on your prostate health. Water enhances chemical reactions, regulates temperature and blood volume and transports waste and nutrients. This can promote prostate health by flushing away toxins that may be lingering within the gland. For conditions such as prostatitis, which causes an enlarged prostate, the University of Maryland Medical Center recommends consumption of 48 ounces of water daily. Additional sources of fluids include fruit juices, vegetables juices and herbal teas

Along with drinking fluids warm water baths can be adopted for prostate natural cures particularly for chronic prostatitis , as these baths will help to deal with the pain by regulating the blood circulation .

Use alternating hot and cold water

For the low abdomen (3 minutes hot and maximum 1 minute cold) ,by either using a shower or splashes in the bath. The ideal method is using Sitz baths, as in hydrotherapy clinics.

 The sitz bath involves filling the bath tub with water to the pelvic region of the body ,up to the navel.

The cold treatment is recommended for the disorder in the pelvic and sacral (of the sacrum) region , such as the prolepses of the rectum and uterus, excess menstrual bleeding, bleeding piles and prostrate problems.

The hot sitz is good for non-bleeding piles, menstrual cramps, urinary infections, Itching of the arms and genitals ,Anal and viginal irritation.

Wet girdle pack should be applied

A wet girdle pack is another valuable remedy in the realm of hydrotherapy, which provides great relief in prostatitis and prostate enlargement. For this mode of treatment, thin cotton underwear and thick or woollen underwear are required. The thin underwear should be wrung in cold water and worn by the patient. The thick dry underwear should be worn above the wet underwear. This treatment should be continued for ninety minute regularly every night. If the patient feels chilly, he should be covered with a blanket.

Treatment of urinary Retention

Urinary retention is a complication associated with prostrate enlargement , benign prostatic hyperplasia (BPH) . It occurs when the gland enlarges to the point where it blocks the flow of urine through the uretha.

A competent Health Provider needs to take an immediate action for the evacuating of the bladder with the aid of a catheter

Catheterization:

The treatment begins with the insertion of a catheter through the urethra to drain the bladder. This initial treatment relieves the immediate distress of a full bladder and prevents permanent bladder damage and other related problems.

The cause of acute urinary retention may be temporary.

Long-term treatment for any case of urinary retention depends on the cause.

The main reason for the use of catheters is for urine collection and to provide access to the bladder.

Occasionally, difficulty can be encountered with the insertion of the catheter due to issues such as an enlarged prostate gland in males, or unusually small urethral opening and/or strictures within the urethra (channel from the bladder to the outside) in both sexes.This can be overcome with the use of correct types by qualified and competent Health Provider.
 The insertion of the catheter is to aid the evacuation of the urine from the bladder while all efforts is concentrated on shrinking the enlarged prostrate.

Dictionary of some Medical Terminologies used.

Listed below in an alphabetical order are some medical/nutritional terminologies used in this book for easy and better understanding of some expressions.

abortifacient - inducing abortion

adjuvant - aiding the action of a medicinal agent

analeptic - restorative or stimulating effect on central nervous system

analgesic - relieve pain

anaphrodisiac - reduces capacity for sexual arousal

anesthetic - induces loss of sensation or consciousness due to the depression of nerve function

antianemic - preventing or curing anemia

antibacterial - destroying or stopping the growth of bacteria

antibilious - easing stomach stress

anticatarrh - reduces inflamed mucous membranes of head and throat

antidepressant - therapy that acts to prevent, cure, or alleviate mental depression

antidiabetic - preventing or relieving diabetes

antidiarrhetic- substances use to prevent or treat diarrhea

antiemetic - stopping vomiting

antifungal - destroying or inhibiting the growth of fungus

antihemorrhagic - controlling hemorrhaging or bleeding

anti-infectous - counteracting infection

anti-inflammatory - controlling inflammation, a reaction to injury or infection

antimalarial - preventing or relieving malaria

antimicrobial - destructive to microbes

antioxident - prevents or inhibits oxidation

antipruritic - preventing or relieving itching

antipyretic - agent that reduces fever (febrifuge)

antirheumatic - easing pain of rheumatism, inflammation of joints and muscles

antiseptic - agent used to produce asepsis and to remove pus, blood, etc.

antispasmodic - calming nervous and muscular spasms or convulsions

antitussive - controlling or preventing cough

antiviral - opposing the action of a virus

aperient - a very mild laxative

aperitive - stimulating the appetite for food

aphrodisiac - substance increasing capacity for sexual arousal

asepsis - sterile, a condition free of germs, infection, and any form of life

astringent - agent that constricts and binds by coagulation of proteins a cell surface

bitter - stimulates appetite or digestive function

cardiotonic - increases strength and tone (normal tension or response to stimuli) of the heart

carminative - causing the release of stomach or intestinal gas

catarrhal - pertaining to the inflammation of mucous membranes of the head and throat

cathartic - an active purgative, producing bowel movements

cholagogue - an agent that increases flow of bile from gallbladder

cicatrizant - aiding formation of scar-tissue and healing wounds

counterirritant - agent producing an inflammatory response for affecting an adjacent area

demulcent - soothing action on inflammation, especially of mucous membranes

dermatitis - inflammation of the skin evidenced my itchiness, redness, and various lesions

diaphoretic - increases perspiration (syn: sudorific)

diuretic - increases urine flow

dysmenorrhea - painful menstruation

dyspepsia - imperfect or painful digestion

ecbolic - tends to increase contractions of uterus, facilitating childbirth

emetic - produces vomiting

emmenagogue - agent that regulates and induces normal menstruation

emollient - softens and soothes the skin

errhine - bringing on sneezing, increasing flow of mucus in nasal passages

escharotic - a caustic substance that destroys tissue and causes sloughing

estrogenic - causes the production of estrogen

euphoriant - produces a sense of bodily comfort; temporary effect and often addictive

expectorant - facilitates removal of secretions

febrifuge - an agent that reduces or relieves a fever

flatulence - excessive gas in the stomach or intestine

galactagogue - an agent that promotes the flow of milk (syn: galactogenic)

hemagogue - an agent that promotes the flow of blood

hemostatic - controls the flow or stops the flow of blood

hepatic - having to do with the liver

herpetic - treating skin eruptions relating to the herpes virus

hypertensive - raises blood pressure

hypoglycemant - agent that lowers blood sugar

hypotensive - lowers blood pressure

lactifuge - reduces the flow of milk

laxative - substance that acts to loosen the bowels contents

masticatory - increases flow of saliva upon chewing

narcotic - induces drowsiness, sleep, or stupor and lessons pain

nervine - a nerve tonic

neuralgia - severe sharp pain along the course of a nerve

parturfaciant - induces contractions of labor at childbirth

purgative - laxative, causes the evacuation of intestinal contents

resorbent - aids reabsorption of blood from bruises

rheumatism - a general term for acute or chronic conditions
characterized by inflammation of the muscles and joints (includes
arthritis, gout, bursitis, myositis, and fibromyositis).

rubefacient - agent which reddens skin, dilates the vessels, and increases blood supply locally

sedative - exerts a soothing, tranquilizing effect on the body

soporific - inducing sleep

stimulant - temporarily increases body or organ function

stomachic - aids the stomach and digestion action

sudorific - acts to increase perspiration

tonic - a substance that increases strength and tone (top)

Medical Terminology

abortifacient - inducing abortion

adjuvant - aiding the action of a medicinal agent

analeptic - restorative or stimulating effect on central nervous system

analgesic - relieve pain

anaphrodisiac - reduces capacity for sexual arousal

anesthetic - induces loss of sensation or consciousness due to the depression of nerve function

antianemic - preventing or curing anemia

antibacterial - destroying or stopping the growth of bacteria

antibilious - easing stomach stress

anticatarrh - reduces inflamed mucous membranes of head and throat

antidepressant - therapy that acts to prevent, cure, or alleviate mental depression

antidiabetic - preventing or relieving diabetes

antidiarrhetic- substances use to prevent or treat diarrhea

antiemetic - stopping vomiting

antifungal - destroying or inhibiting the growth of fungus

antihemorrhagic - controlling hemorrhaging or bleeding

anti-infectous - counteracting infection

anti-inflammatory - controlling inflammation, a reaction to injury or infection

antimalarial - preventing or relieving malaria

antimicrobial - destructive to microbes

antioxident - prevents or inhibits oxidation

antipruritic - preventing or relieving itching

antipyretic - agent that reduces fever (febrifuge)

antirheumatic - easing pain of rheumatism, inflammation of joints and muscles

antiseptic - agent used to produce asepsis and to remove pus, blood, etc.

antispasmodic - calming nervous and muscular spasms or convulsions

antitussive - controlling or preventing cough

antiviral - opposing the action of a virus

aperient - a very mild laxative

aperitive - stimulating the appetite for food

aphrodisiac - substance increasing capacity for sexual arousal

asepsis - sterile, a condition free of germs, infection, and any form of life

astringent - agent that constricts and binds by coagulation of proteins a cell surface

bitter - stimulates appetite or digestive function

cardiotonic - increases strength and tone (normal tension or response to stimuli) of the heart

carminative - causing the release of stomach or intestinal gas catarrhal - pertaining to the inflammation of mucous membranes of the head and throat

cathartic - an active purgative, producing bowel movements

cholagogue - an agent that increases flow of bile from gallbladder

cicatrizant - aiding formation of scar-tissue and healing wounds

counterirritant - agent producing an inflammatory response for affecting an adjacent area

demulcent - soothing action on inflammation, especially of mucous membranes

dermatitis - inflammation of the skin evidenced my itchiness, redness, and various lesions

diaphoretic - increases perspiration (syn: sudorific)

diuretic - increases urine flow

dysmenorrhea - painful menstruation

dyspepsia - imperfect or painful digestion

ecbolic - tends to increase contractions of uterus, facilitating childbirth

emetic - produces vomiting

emmenagogue - agent that regulates and induces normal menstruation

emollient - softens and soothes the skin

errhine - bringing on sneezing, increasing flow of mucus in nasal passages

escharotic - a caustic substance that destroys tissue and causes sloughing

estrogenic - causes the production of estrogen

euphoriant - produces a sense of bodily comfort; temporary effect and often addictive

expectorant - facilitates removal of secretions

febrifuge - an agent that reduces or relieves a fever

flatulence - excessive gas in the stomach or intestine

galactagogue - an agent that promotes the flow of milk (syn: galactogenic)

hemagogue - an agent that promotes the flow of blood

hemostatic - controls the flow or stops the flow of blood

hepatic - having to do with the liver

herpetic - treating skin eruptions relating to the herpes virus hypertensive - raises blood pressure

hypoglycemant - agent that lowers blood sugar

hypotensive - lowers blood pressure

lactifuge - reduces the flow of milk

laxative - substance that acts to loosen the bowels contents

masticatory - increases flow of saliva upon chewing

narcotic - induces drowsiness, sleep, or stupor and lessons pain

nervine - a nerve tonic

neuralgia - severe sharp pain along the course of a nerve

parturfaciant - induces contractions of labor at childbirth

purgative - laxative, causes the evacuation of intestinal contents

resorbent - aids reabsorption of blood from bruises

rheumatism - a general term for acute or chronic conditions characterized by inflammation of the muscles and joints (includes arthritis, gout, bursitis, myositis, and fibromyositis).

rubefacient - agent which reddens skin, dilates the vessels, and increases blood supply locally

sedative - exerts a soothing, tranquilizing effect on the body

soporific - inducing sleep

stimulant - temporarily increases body or organ function

stomachic - aids the stomach and digestion action

sudorific - acts to increase perspiration

tonic - a substance that increases strength and tone (top